I0790272

Also by Chris Josinlah

The Minimalist Monk's Guide to a Clutter-Free Life: Zen Approach to a Tidy Home & Mind
Age Well, Live Fully: Your Mind-Body Prescription

Table of Contents

Introduction

Age, like a river, carries us inexorably forward. Its current is steady, its direction unyielding. Yet, unlike a river, we possess the capacity to shape its course. We can navigate the rapids, find solace in its calm stretches, and even alter its flow. This is the essence of aging well.

It is a journey often painted with hues of decline, a descent into a twilight existence. But this is a misconception, a shadow cast by societal stereotypes. The reality is far more vibrant, a tapestry woven with threads of resilience, wisdom, and growth.

At the heart of aging well there is a profound connection between mind and body—an intricate dance of interdependence. Our thoughts, emotions, and beliefs shape our physical experiences, while our bodies, in turn, influence our mental state. It is this symbiotic relationship that holds the key to unlocking a fulfilling later life.

To age well is not merely to survive, but to thrive. It is to face the inevitable challenges of aging with courage, to discover new passions, and to cultivate a sense of purpose. It is to embrace change as an opportunity for growth, rather than a threat to our identity.

This book, **Age Well, Live Fully: Your Mind-Body Prescription**, is an invitation to embark upon a transformative journey. It is a guide to navigating the complexities of aging, a roadmap to unlocking the full potential of your mind and body. Let us explore together the possibilities that await us as we traverse the later chapters of life.

Are you ready to rewrite the script on aging?

Aging is not a destination but a journey. It is a chapter filled with unique challenges and extraordinary opportunities. This book offers a comprehensive guide to navigating this journey with grace, resilience, and vitality.

Throughout these pages, you will discover the intricate relationship between mind and body, and how this connection can profoundly influence your overall well-being. We will explore the key principles for aging well, including nourishing your body, moving your mind, and cultivating a supportive environment.

This book is more than just information. It is a practical guide, filled with actionable advice and exercises to help you implement these principles in your daily life.

Whether you're seeking to improve your physical health, enhance your mental clarity, or simply find more joy in your later years, this book will provide the tools and strategies you need.

Let's embark on this journey together, unlocking the full potential of your mind and body as you age gracefully.

Chapter 1: Comprehending the Mind-Body Connection

The Science Behind the Mind-Body Relationship

For centuries, philosophers and mystics pondered the intricate dance between mind and body. Today, science is beginning to unravel the complex network that bind these two realms. Our thoughts, emotions, and beliefs are not mere abstractions but potent forces that shape our physical reality.

The brain, once considered a solitary organ, is now understood as a command center in constant communication with the body. Every sensation, every emotion, every thought triggers a cascade of biochemical reactions that ripple through our physiology.

Our nervous system, the body's communication network, carries messages back and forth, ensuring a seamless interplay between mind and body.

The Impact of Stress on the Body

Stress, an unwelcome companion in modern life, is a prime example of the mind-body relationship in action.

When faced with perceived threats, our bodies activate a fight-or-flight response, flooding the system with stress hormones. While this reaction was essential for our survival in the face of predators, chronic stress can wreak havoc on our health.

High levels of cortisol, the primary stress hormone, can weaken the immune system, increase blood pressure, disrupt sleep patterns, and contribute to a host of chronic diseases.

Moreover, stress can exacerbate existing conditions and accelerate the aging process. It's a stark reminder of the profound impact our mental state can have on our physical well-being.

The Role of Emotions in Physical Health

Emotions are the language of the soul, expressed through the body. Joy, love, and gratitude can uplift our spirits and strengthen our immune system. Conversely, anger, fear, and sadness can create physical tension, inflammation, and even disease.

The field of psychoneuroimmunology has revealed the intricate link between emotions and the immune system. Positive emotions can stimulate the production of antibodies, while negative emotions can suppress immune function. Our bodies are exquisitely attuned to our emotional landscape, and the health of one directly influences the other.

The Role of Humor and Laughter

Laughter is a powerful tool for boosting mood, reducing stress, and strengthening the immune system. Incorporating humor into your daily life can help you maintain a positive outlook and improve your overall well-being.

Practical Tip: Watch a funny movie, read a humorous book, or spend time with people who make you laugh.

The Lesser Known Importance of Emotional Intelligence

Emotional intelligence, often overlooked, is the ability to understand and manage our own emotions as well as those of others. It involves self-awareness, empathy, and effective communication. By cultivating emotional intelligence, we can improve our relationships, make sound decisions, and navigate life's challenges with greater resilience. This often-overlooked skill is a cornerstone of mental well-being.

Practical Exercise: Gratitude Journaling

1. Find an designated notebook: This can be a physical journal or a digital document.
2. Write down three things you're grateful for: Each day, take a few minutes to reflect on the positive aspects of your life.

3. Be specific: The more detailed your entries, the greater the impact.
4. Reflect regularly: Aim to practice gratitude journaling daily or at least a few times a week.

Gratitude journaling can shift your focus towards the positive, reducing stress and improving your overall well-being. By acknowledging the good things in your life, you can cultivate a more optimistic mindset and foster resilience.

Power of the Placebo Effect

The mind holds incredible power over the body, as shown by the placebo effect. A seemingly inert substance, when administered with conviction, can produce remarkable healing effects. This phenomenon highlights the role of belief and expectation in shaping our physical reality.

While the exact mechanisms remain a subject of scientific inquiry, it is clear that our minds can influence physiological processes at a profound level.

The placebo effect underscores the importance of hope, optimism, and a positive outlook in the healing process.

The Power of Mindfulness

Mindfulness, the practice of being present in the moment, is a powerful tool for improving mental and physical health. By focusing our attention on the present moment, we can reduce stress, increase self-awareness, and cultivate a sense of inner peace. Mindfulness techniques, such as meditation and deep breathing, can help us connect with our bodies and minds on a deeper level.

Mindfulness is not just a buzzword; it's a scientifically proven practice that can significantly impact our mental and physical health. Neuroimaging studies have shown that mindfulness meditation can increase brain activity in areas associated with attention, awareness, and emotional regulation.

Practical Exercise: Mindful Meditation

1. Find a quiet space: Sit or lie down comfortably, closing your eyes.
2. Focus on your breath: Pay attention to the sensation of your breath as

it enters and exits your body.

3. Observe without judgment: Notice any thoughts or feelings that arise, but don't dwell on them. Simply return your attention to your breath.
4. Practice for 5-10 minutes: Gradually increase the duration as you become more comfortable.

This simple exercise can help you cultivate mindfulness, reduce stress, and deepen your understanding of the mind-body connection. By focusing on your breath, you'll become more aware of your physical sensations and emotional state.

The Role of Yoga and Meditation

Yoga and meditation are ancient practices that have been shown to have numerous benefits for physical and mental health. Yoga combines physical postures, breathing exercises, and meditation to promote flexibility, strength, and relaxation. Meditation, on the other hand, involves training the mind to focus and redirect thoughts.

Practical Exercise: Yoga Nidra

1. Find a quiet place to lie down.
2. Close your eyes and focus on your breath.
3. Gradually relax each part of your body, starting with your toes and working your way up to your head.
4. Visualize a peaceful scene and focus on your breath.
5. Practice for 10-20 minutes each day.

The Impact of Breathwork on Mental Health

Breathwork is a powerful technique that involves conscious breathing exercises to improve physical and mental health. By regulating our breath, we can influence our heart rate, blood pressure, and stress levels. Deep, slow breathing can calm the nervous system, reduce anxiety, depression, stress, and improve focus. Breathwork techniques, such as diaphragmatic breathing and pranayama, can have a profound impact on mental health.

Practical Exercise: Diaphragmatic Breathing

1. Find a comfortable position, such as sitting or lying down.
2. Place one hand on your chest and the other on your stomach.
3. Inhale slowly and deeply, allowing your stomach to rise.
4. Exhale slowly, drawing your stomach inward.
5. Practice for 5-10 minutes each day.

Chapter 2: Biohacking Secrets

Biohacking is a cutting-edge field that empowers individuals to take control of their health and performance. By optimizing your body and mind through evidence-based strategies, comprehending the underlying mechanisms of health and well-being, we can implement strategies to enhance cognitive function, physical performance, and overall quality of life.

In this chapter, we'll explore some key biohacking techniques that can complement your aging journey. Remember, while biohacking offers exciting possibilities, it's important to consult with a healthcare professional before making significant changes to your lifestyle or health regimen.

Sleep Optimization

Create a relaxing bedtime routine to ensure a comfortable sleep environment. Sleep tracking devices can provide valuable insights into your sleep patterns, including sleep duration, sleep stages, and sleep quality. By monitoring your sleep, you can identify areas for improvement and make adjustments to your lifestyle to optimize your rest.

The Benefits of Sleep Tracking:

- Improved cognitive function

- Enhanced mood

- Boosted immune system

- Increased energy levels

- Reduced risk of chronic diseases

Blue Light Shield

How Does Blue Light Affect Your Body?

Exposure to blue light, emitted by electronic devices, can disrupt your sleep-wake cycle, leading to difficulty falling asleep and poor sleep quality.

How Can the Blue Light Exposure Problem Be Resolved?

- **Use Night Shift Mode:** Activate night shift mode on your devices to reduce blue light emission.

- **Wear Blue Light Blocking Glasses:** These glasses can help filter out harmful blue light.

- **Limit Screen Time Before Bed:** Avoid using electronic devices for at least an hour before bedtime.

The Power of Alkaline Water:

Why is Alkaline Water Better?

Alkaline water has a higher pH level than regular water, which can help neutralize acidity in the body. Some studies suggest that alkaline water may have several health benefits, including improved digestion, increased energy levels, and reduced inflammation.

Harnessing the Power of Red Light Therapy:

What is Red Light Therapy?

Red light therapy involves exposing your skin to specific wavelengths of red and near-infrared light. This therapy has gained popularity for its potential benefits for skin health, muscle recovery, and pain relief.

How to Benefit from Red Light Therapy:

- **Skin Health:** Red light therapy can help reduce wrinkles, improve skin texture, and promote collagen production.

- **Muscle Recovery:** It can accelerate muscle recovery and reduce inflammation.

- **Pain Relief:** Red light therapy may help alleviate pain associated with conditions like arthritis and fibromyalgia.

The Importance of Physical Activity:

The Problems of a Sedentary Lifestyle

A sedentary lifestyle can lead to a host of health problems, including obesity, heart disease, and diabetes.

How Can I Get More Active?

- Incorporate Exercise into Your Routine: Find activities you enjoy, such as walking, running, cycling, or swimming.

- Set Realistic Goals: Start with small, achievable goals and gradually increase the intensity and duration of your workouts.

- Find a Workout Buddy: Having a workout partner can help you stay motivated and accountable.

The Practice of Mindfulness

Mindfulness is the practice of being present in the moment. It involves paying attention to your thoughts, feelings, and sensations without judgment.

How Does Mindfulness Work?

Mindfulness can reduce stress, anxiety, and depression. It can also improve focus, memory, and overall well-being.

Top Tips for Introducing Mindfulness Practice into Your Life:

- **Mindful Breathing:** Focus on your breath, inhaling and exhaling slowly and deeply.

- **Meditation:** Practice meditation for 5-30 minutes each day.

- **Mindful Eating**: Pay attention to the taste, smell, and texture of your food.

The Power of Whole Foods:

The Junk Food Problem

Consuming processed foods high in sugar, unhealthy fats, and artificial additives can negatively impact your health.

What Are Whole Foods?

Whole foods are minimally processed foods that retain their natural nutrients. They include fruits, vegetables, whole grains, lean proteins, and healthy fats.

Why Eat More Whole Foods?

- Improved digestion

- Boosted immune system

- Increased energy levels

- Reduced risk of chronic diseases

How to Eat More Whole Foods:

- **Plan your meals:** Create a weekly meal plan to ensure you're eating balanced meals.

- **Cook at home:** Prepare your own meals to control the ingredients and avoid processed foods.

- **Snack smart:** Choose healthy snacks like fruits, vegetables, and nuts.

The Gut-Brain Connection and Probiotics

What Exactly Are Probiotics?

Probiotics are live bacteria that can benefit your gut health. A healthy gut microbiome is essential for overall well-being, including mental health.

How to Incorporate Probiotics into Your Diet:

- **Consume fermented foods:** Yogurt, kefir, sauerkraut, and kimchi are excellent sources of probiotics.

- **Take probiotic supplements:** Consult with a healthcare professional to determine the best probiotic supplement for your needs.

Cryotherapy: A New Frontier in Wellness

What is Cryotherapy?

Cryotherapy involves exposure to extremely cold temperatures for a short period. It's believed to have numerous health benefits, including reduced inflammation, improved muscle recovery, and enhanced mood.

What are the Benefits of Cryotherapy?

- **Pain relief:** Cryotherapy can help alleviate pain associated with conditions like arthritis and fibromyalgia.

- **Improved athletic performance**: It can help reduce muscle soreness and accelerate recovery time.

- **Enhanced mood:** Cryotherapy may help improve mood and reduce symptoms of depression and anxiety.

By incorporating biohacking techniques into your daily routine, you can take control of your health and well-being. Remember, it's essential to listen to your body and make adjustments as needed. While biohacking offers exciting possibilities, it's crucial to approach it with a balanced and sustainable mindset.

By combining the wisdom of ancient practices like mindfulness and meditation with cutting-edge biohacking techniques, you can unlock your full potential and age gracefully.

Chapter 3: Peace and Joy Through Self-Care

Self-Care Using CBT and Mindfulness

Cognitive Behavioral Therapy (CBT) is a form of psychotherapy that helps people understand and change their thought patterns. By identifying and challenging negative thoughts, individuals can reduce anxiety, depression, and other mental health issues.

Mindfulness, on the other hand, is the practice of being present in the moment, without judgment. It can help reduce stress, improve focus, and enhance overall well-being.

Silencing the Inner Critic

- **Mindfulness:** Mindfulness meditation is a powerful tool for silencing the inner critic. By focusing on the present moment, you can observe your thoughts without judgment. This can help you to identify negative thought patterns and challenge them.

- **Positive Self-Talk:** Replace negative self-talk with positive affirmations. Remind yourself of your strengths, accomplishments, and positive qualities.

- **Hypothesis Testing:** Question the validity of your negative thoughts. Are they based on facts or assumptions? By challenging negative thoughts, you can reframe your perspective and reduce self-doubt.

Self-Fulfilling Prophecies

The Law of Attraction: The law of attraction suggests that positive thoughts attract positive experiences. By focusing on positive outcomes, you can manifest your desires.

Practical Tips:

- **Visualize Success:** Imagine yourself achieving your goals.

- **Affirm Positive Beliefs:** Repeat positive affirmations daily.

- **Practice Gratitude:** Focus on the positive aspects of your life.

Looking After Your Looks:

It's the Little Things:

- **Posture:** Good posture can make you look and feel more confident.

- **Smile:** A smile can brighten your day and the days of those around you.

- **Eye Contact:** Make eye contact to show that you're engaged and interested.

How to Beam:

- **Radiate Positivity:** Positive energy is contagious.

- **Dress Well:** Choose clothing that makes you feel good about yourself.

- **Practice Good Hygiene:** Take care of your personal hygiene to feel and look your best.

Putting On Your Best Face:

- **Skincare Routine:** Develop a daily skincare routine that suits your skin type.

- **Hair Care:** Keep your hair clean, styled, and healthy.

- **Makeup Tips:** If you so choose, use makeup to enhance your natural beauty.

Grooming:

- **Regular Grooming:** Maintain your nails, eyebrows, and other areas as needed.

- **Fragrance:** Choose a fragrance that complements your personality.

Taking Care of Your Health:

Getting Started with a Fitness Regime:

- **Start Slowly:** Begin with low-impact exercises like walking or swimming.

- **Find a Workout Buddy:** Having a workout partner can help you stay motivated.

- **Set Realistic Goals:** Start with small, achievable goals and gradually increase the intensity and duration of your workouts.

Letting Go of Regrets:

Do Regrets Fade With Time?

While time can help to soften the sting of regrets, it's important to address them in a healthy way.

That Which Has Been Done...

- **Accept the Past:** Acknowledge your past mistakes and learn from them.

- **Focus on the Present:** Shift your attention to the present moment.

- **Practice Forgiveness:** Forgive yourself and others for past mistakes.

The Power of Gratitude and Self-Compassion:

Loving-Kindness Meditation and Gratitude:

- **Practice Gratitude**: Regularly express gratitude for the good things in your life.

- **Cultivate Self-Compassion**: Treat yourself with kindness and understanding.

Say Goodbye to Social Anxiety:

Use CBT and Become Socially Bulletproof:

- **Challenge Negative Thoughts**: Identify and challenge negative thoughts about social situations.

- **Practice Social Skills**: Start with small interactions and gradually increase your social exposure.

- **Exposure Therapy**: Gradually expose yourself to social situations that make you anxious.

Changing Your Environment:

Awe and Wonder:

Spend Time in Nature: Connect with nature to reduce stress and boost your mood.

Practice Mindfulness in Nature: Pay attention to the sights, sounds, and smells of the natural world.

The Healing Power of Nature:

Gardening: Gardening can be a therapeutic and rewarding activity.

Forest Bathing: Spend time in a forest or other natural setting.

Your Home:

Declutter Your Space: A clutter-free environment can promote peace and tranquility.

Create a Cozy Retreat: Design a space where you can relax and recharge.

Why There's Really No Need for Low-Self Esteem:

Embrace Your Uniqueness: Recognize your strengths and celebrate your individuality.

Practice Self-Compassion: Treat yourself with kindness and understanding.

Challenge Negative Beliefs: Replace negative thoughts with positive affirmations.

Set Realistic Goals: Break down large goals into smaller, achievable steps.

Celebrate Your Achievements: Acknowledge and appreciate your successes, no matter how small.

Your Blueprint for Living Fully Through Self-Care

By incorporating these strategies into your daily life, you can improve your mental, physical and emotional well-being. Remember, self-care is an ongoing process. Be patient with yourself and celebrate your progress.

Chapter 4: Environmental Factors and Aging

The Impact of Climate Change on Aging

Climate change poses significant risks to older adults, who are more vulnerable to the effects of extreme weather events, such as heatwaves and cold spells. Air pollution can exacerbate respiratory and cardiovascular conditions, further impacting the health of older adults.

Practical Tips:

Stay informed: Stay updated on weather forecasts and health advisories.

Create a safe indoor environment: Ensure your home is well-insulated and air-conditioned.

Check on neighbors and loved ones: Offer assistance to those who may be more vulnerable.

Creating Age-Friendly Environments

Age-friendly communities are designed to meet the needs of older adults and promote healthy aging. These communities offer accessible housing, transportation, and healthcare services.

Practical Tips:

- **Modify your home:** Make necessary modifications to your home, such as installing grab bars and ramps.

- **Use assistive devices:** Utilize assistive devices like canes, walkers, or wheelchairs to improve mobility.

- **Get involved in community planning:** Advocate for age-friendly policies and infrastructure.

The Role of Green Spaces

Spending time in nature has numerous benefits for physical and mental health. Green spaces can reduce stress, improve mood, and boost the immune system.

Practical Tips:

Spend time outdoors: Engage in activities like gardening, walking, or simply sitting in a park.

Bring nature indoors: Incorporate plants into your home to improve air quality and create a calming atmosphere.

Support local initiatives to protect green spaces: Volunteer or donate to organizations that work to preserve nature.

Chapter 5: Unlocking Youthful Vitality: The Science of Optimizing Longevity

This chapter will delve deeper into the science behind aging and explore specific strategies to slow down the aging process.

Comprehending the Aging Process

Aging is a complex process influenced by a variety of factors, including genetics, lifestyle, and environmental factors. As we age, our cells undergo changes that can lead to wrinkles, age spots, and decreased muscle mass. However, by adopting healthy habits and lifestyle modifications, we can slow down the aging process and maintain a youthful appearance.

Key Strategies for Timeless Elegance

Sun Protection:

- Wear sunscreen daily, even on cloudy days.
- Seek shade during peak sun hours.
- Wear protective clothing, such as hats and sunglasses.

Nutrition: Cellular Longevity Boosters

Polyphenol-Rich Diet: Focus on foods like dark chocolate, olive oil, and berries. Polyphenols combat oxidative stress and have an anti-inflammatory effect.

Intermittent Fasting Variations: Less common variations, like the 16:8 method, have been shown to stimulate autophagy (cellular cleansing) and could support cellular repair.

Healthy Nutrition:

- Ingest produce rich in fruits, vegetables, whole grains, and lean protein.

- Limit processed foods, sugary drinks, and excessive amounts of saturated and unhealthy fats.

- Stay hydrated by drinking plenty of water.

Movement and Flexibility Practices

Functional Movement Exercises: Integrate full-range movements to maintain muscle and joint health - this could include dynamic stretching, yoga-inspired poses, or Pilates routines.

Practical Exercise: A 5-minute morning mobility sequence that keeps joints fluid and helps prevent stiffness.

Regular Exercise:

Engage in a variety of physical activities, including cardiovascular exercise, strength training, and flexibility exercises.

Aim for at least 30 minutes of moderate-intensity exercise most days of the week.

Mindfulness and Brain Health:

Artistic Hobbies for Brain Longevity: Engaging in creative pursuits like painting or music can stimulate neuroplasticity, helping to maintain cognitive flexibility.

Meditative Walks: Combine walking with mindfulness practices to increase blood flow to the brain while reducing stress.

Quality Sleep:

Prioritize 7-9 hours of quality sleep each night.

Create a relaxing bedtime routine to wind down before sleep.

Optimize your sleep environment for darkness, quiet, and a comfortable temperature.

Stress Resilience and Hormonal Balance:

Forest Bathing (Shinrin-Yoku): Spending time in nature, specifically around trees, is shown to reduce cortisol and boost immune function, enhancing longevity.

Breathwork for Cortisol Control: Practice a simple breathing technique (e.g., 4-7-8 breath) for 5 minutes daily to reset the nervous system and minimize stress-induced aging.

Stress Management:

Practice stress-reduction techniques like meditation, yoga, or deep breathing.

Manage stress through time management, setting boundaries, and seeking support from loved ones.

Skincare Beyond the Surface

Microbiome-Friendly Products: Opt for skincare that nurtures your skin's microbiome to support natural immunity and resilience. Use products with probiotics, prebiotics, and gentle formulations.

Facial Acupressure: Practical exercise: a daily 5-minute routine of pressing key points to relieve tension and promote circulation for a natural glow.

Skincare Routine:

Cleanse your face twice daily.

Use a gentle moisturizer to keep your skin hydrated.

Apply sunscreen daily.

Consider using anti-aging products with ingredients like retinol, vitamin C, and hyaluronic acid.

By incorporating these strategies into your daily routine, you can slow down the aging process and maintain a youthful appearance. Remember, consistency is key. Small changes can lead to significant results over time.

Chapter 6: Moving Your Body

Exercise for All Ages and Fitness Levels

Movement is the elixir of youth, a potent antidote to the ravages of time. Physical activity is not merely a means to burn calories or sculpt muscles; it is a cornerstone of holistic health. Regardless of age or fitness level, there is a form of exercise that can enhance quality of life. Whether it's a brisk walk, gentle yoga, or a vigorous dance class, finding joy in movement is key.

The Role of Physical Activity in Cognitive Health

Regular physical activity has been shown to improve cognitive function, including memory, attention, and problem-solving skills. Exercise stimulates the production of brain-derived neurotrophic factor (BDNF), a protein that promotes the growth and survival of brain cells.

Practical Tip: Aim for at least 30 minutes of moderate-intensity exercise most days of the week.

Strength Training for Longevity

Building muscle mass is often associated with youth, but its importance endures as we age. Strength training not only tones the body but also strengthens bones, preventing osteoporosis and reducing the risk of fractures. It improves balance, coordination, and overall functional capacity, empowering individuals to maintain independence well into their later years..

Practical Tip: Incorporate strength training exercises, such as lifting weights or using resistance bands, into your weekly routine.

Low-Impact Exercises

Low-impact exercises, such as Yoga, Pilates, and Tai Chi, are gentle on the joints and can be beneficial for people of all ages. These activities improve flexibility, balance, and coordination, reducing the risk of falls and injuries.

Practical Tip: Find a class or online video that suits your fitness level and preferences.

The Importance of Flexibility and Balance

As we age, our bodies naturally become less flexible. Maintaining a good range of motion is crucial for preventing injuries, improving posture, and enhancing daily activities. Yoga, Pilates, and Tai Chi are also excellent modalities for cultivating flexibility. Balance, too, is a vital component of aging well. Exercises that challenge our equilibrium, such as standing on one leg or walking heel-to-toe, can significantly reduce the risk of falls.

The Benefits of Outdoor Exercise

Nature has a profound impact on our well-being. Engaging in outdoor activities not only provides physical benefits but also reduces stress, improves mood, and connects us with the natural world. Whether it's gardening, hiking, or simply taking a walk in the park, spending time outdoors can rejuvenate the body and mind.

The Lesser Known Role of Proprioceptive Exercises

Proprioception, the body's sense of spatial orientation, is essential for balance, coordination, and injury prevention. Engaging in activities that challenge this sense can improve overall physical performance and reduce the risk of falls. Exercises like standing on unstable surfaces, balancing on one leg with eyes closed, and performing plyometric movements can enhance proprioception.

The Role of Yoga and Meditation in Combating Chronic Pain

Chronic pain can significantly impact quality of life. Yoga and meditation have been shown to be effective in managing chronic pain. Yoga poses can help to improve flexibility, strength, and balance, while meditation can help to reduce pain perception and promote relaxation.

Practical Tips: Yoga for Pain Relief

- **Gentle Yoga:** Start with gentle yoga poses that focus on stretching and relaxation.

- **Mindful Movement:** Pay attention to your body's sensations and adjust your practice accordingly.

- **Breathwork:** Incorporate deep breathing exercises to enhance relaxation and pain relief.

Practical Exercise: Chair Yoga

1. **Find a comfortable chair:** Ensure it has a firm back and armrests.
2. **Start with gentle stretches:** Reach for the sky, twist your torso, and circle your shoulders.
3. **Strengthen your legs:** Perform chair squats, leg raises, and ankle circles.
4. **Improve balance:** Practice standing on one leg for short intervals.
5. **Relax your body:** Finish with deep breathing and relaxation techniques.

Chair yoga is a gentle form of exercise that can be done from the comfort of your home. It's suitable for all fitness levels and can help improve flexibility, strength, balance, and reduce stress.

Chapter 7: Decluttering and Minimalism

Why Declutter?

Decluttering isn't just about organizing your space; it's about decluttering your mind. A cluttered environment can lead to stress, anxiety, and difficulty focusing. By decluttering, you're creating a more peaceful and organized living space, which can have a positive impact on your mental and emotional well-being.

The Benefits of Decluttering:

1. **Reduced Stress:** A clutter-free environment can reduce stress and anxiety.
2. **Increased Productivity:** A clutter-free workspace can improve focus and productivity.
3. **Improved Mental Health:** Decluttering can boost your mood and reduce feelings of overwhelm.
4. **Financial Freedom:** Decluttering can help you save money by reducing unnecessary purchases.

Practical Tips for Decluttering:

- **Start Small**: Begin by decluttering a small area, such as a drawer or a shelf.

- **Sort and Categorize:** Sort your belongings into three categories: keep, donate, and trash.

- **Be Ruthless:** Don't hold onto items out of sentimentality or guilt.

- **Digital Declutter:** Organize your digital files and delete unnecessary items.

- **Maintain Your Progress:** Regularly declutter to prevent clutter from accumulating.

The Minimalist Lifestyle:

Minimalism is a lifestyle philosophy that emphasizes simplicity and focus. By owning fewer possessions, you can reduce stress, save money, and increase your overall well-being.

Practical Tips for Minimalist Living:

- **Conscious Consumption:** Buy only what you need and avoid impulse purchases.

- **Digital Minimalism:** Limit your screen time and focus on meaningful activities.

- **Mindful Living:** Practice mindfulness to appreciate the simple things in life.

Chapter 8: Technology and Aging

Digital Literacy: Bridging the Gap

In today's digital age, digital literacy is essential for older adults to stay connected, informed, and independent. It empowers individuals to navigate the online world, access information, and communicate with others.

Practical Tips:

- **Start small:** Begin with basic tasks like sending emails and using search engines.

- **Join online communities**: Connect with others who share your interests and learn from their experiences.

- **Take online courses:** Many websites and platforms offer free or low-cost online courses on various topics.

- **Practice regularly:** The more you practice, the more comfortable you'll become with technology.

Social Media and Online Communities

Social media platforms can be a great way to stay connected with friends and family, share interests, and learn new things. However, it's important to be aware of potential pitfalls, such as time-wasting, cyberbullying and misinformation.

Practical Tips:

Choose your platforms wisely: Select platforms that align with your interests and goals.

Be mindful of privacy settings: Protect your personal information by adjusting your privacy settings.

Engage in positive online communities: Join groups that promote kindness, respect, and understanding.

Be cautious of scams and phishing attempts: Avoid clicking on suspicious links or sharing personal information.

Telehealth and Remote Healthcare

Telehealth services offer convenient and accessible healthcare options for older adults, especially those with mobility limitations. These services allow patients to consult with healthcare providers remotely, saving time and reducing the need for in-person visits.

Practical Tips:

Choose a reputable telehealth provider: Research and select a provider that meets your needs.

Prepare for your telehealth appointment: Have a list of questions ready and a reliable internet connection.

Communicate effectively with your healthcare provider: Be clear and concise when explaining your symptoms and concerns.

Use telehealth for preventive care: Schedule regular check-ups and consultations with your healthcare provider.

* * *

Thank you so much for making it this far!

I greatly value the time you're sharing with my book. As a small Indie publisher it means a lot, and I hope I'm making a difference in your Aging Well Journey.

If you have 60 seconds, reading your honest feedback on the site you got it from, would mean the world to me! It does wonders for the book, and I love learning about your experience with it.

So if you're having a positive experience with **Age Well, Live Fully: Your Mind-Body Prescription,** please take a moment to leave a review. Your feedback helps me to improve, and serve more patrons like you.

Chris

***

Chapter 9: Nourishing Your Body

The Importance of Nutrition for Aging Well

Nutrition is the cornerstone of health, and its significance becomes even more pronounced as we age. Our bodies undergo subtle yet profound changes, altering our nutritional needs. What sustained us in our youth may not be optimal for our later years. A diet rich in essential nutrients not only fuels our bodies but also supports cognitive function, immune health, and overall vitality.

Building a Balanced Nutrition Plan

A balanced ingestion plan involves a mosaic of diverse foods, each adding its unique set of nutrients. It's not about strict limitations or fad diets but rather an integrated blend of macronutrients and micronutrients. Prioritizing whole, unprocessed foods forms the foundation of a healthy eating plan. Incorporating a variety of fruits, vegetables, lean proteins, whole grains, and healthy fats ensures that our bodies receive the essential building blocks for optimal function.

Hydration: The Elixir of Life

Often overlooked, hydration is paramount for overall well-being. Water is the solvent for countless bodily processes, from digestion to temperature regulation. As we age, our sense of thirst can diminish, making dehydration a potential risk. Consuming adequate water throughout the day is essential for maintaining energy levels, preventing constipation, and supporting cognitive function. Hydration is essential for optimal health and longevity. Water helps to regulate body temperature, transport nutrients, and eliminate waste products. As we age, our sense of thirst may diminish, making it even more important to stay hydrated.

Practical Tip: Keep a reusable water bottle with you throughout the day and sip water regularly.

The Lesser Known Benefits of Intermittent Fasting

Intermittent fasting, an eating pattern that cycles between periods of eating and fasting, has gained popularity in recent years. While more research is needed, some studies suggest potential benefits for weight management, insulin sensitivity, and cellular repair. It's essential to approach intermittent fasting with caution, especially for individuals with certain health conditions. Consulting with a healthcare professional is advisable before embarking on this dietary pattern.

Practical Exercise: Mindful Eating

1. **Choose a quiet space:** Sit down at a table without distractions.
2. **Focus on your food:** Examine the colors, textures, and aromas of your meal.
3. **Take small bites:** Chew slowly and savor each bite.
4. **Notice the sensations:** Pay attention to the taste, temperature, and texture of the food.
5. **Eat without distractions:** Avoid eating while watching TV, working, or scrolling through your phone.

Mindful eating can help you nurture a healthier relationship with food, appreciate the flavors and textures of your meals, and prevent overeating. By slowing down and paying attention to your body's cues, you can make more mindful choices and nourish your body effectively.

Practical Exercise: Mindful Eating Journal

1. **Track your meals:** Record everything you eat and drink throughout the day.
2. **Note your emotions:** Pay attention to your mood and any emotional triggers that might influence your eating habits.
3. **Observe your body's cues:** Notice feelings of hunger, fullness, and satisfaction.
4. **Reflect on your patterns:** Analyze your journal entries to identify any unhealthy eating habits or emotional eating triggers.

By keeping a mindful eating journal, you can gain valuable insights into your relationship with food and make informed choices to support your gut health and mental well-being. This exercise can help you identify any emotional eating patterns, make healthier food choices, and cultivate a more mindful approach to eating.

The Mediterranean Diet and Longevity

The Mediterranean diet, characterized by its emphasis on plant-based foods, healthy fats, and moderate protein intake, has been linked to numerous health benefits, including longevity. This diet is rich in fruits, vegetables, whole grains, legumes, nuts, and olive oil. It also includes moderate amounts of fish, poultry, and dairy products.

Practical Tip: Incorporate more plant-based meals into your diet. Experiment with different recipes and flavors to keep your meals interesting.

Supplements and Superfoods

While balanced nutrition is the foundation of good health, some individuals may benefit from additional supplementation. Certain vitamins, minerals, and antioxidants may support healthy aging. However, it's important to consult with a healthcare professional before starting any new supplements.

Practical Tip: Incorporate superfoods like berries, leafy green vegetables, and nuts into your diet.

Chapter 10: Lifestyle Factors and Gut Health

The Lesser Known Role of Gut Health in Aging

Emerging research highlights the pivotal role of gut health in aging well. Our intestines are home to trillions of microorganisms collectively known as the gut microbiome. This complex ecosystem influences digestion, immunity, and even brain function. As we age, the composition of the gut microbiome can shift, affecting overall health. Consuming fermented foods, probiotics, and prebiotics can help nurture a thriving gut microbiome, supporting both physical and mental well-being.

The Stress-Gut Connection

The human body is a finely tuned orchestra, and stress is the conductor that can throw it off key. When we're stressed, our bodies release a cascade of hormones, including cortisol, which can disrupt the delicate balance of the gut microbiome. Chronic stress has been linked to conditions like irritable bowel syndrome (IBS) and inflammatory bowel disease (IBD). Managing stress through techniques like meditation, yoga, or deep breathing can significantly benefit gut health.

Sleep and the Gut Microbiome

Sleep, often overlooked as a crucial component of overall well-being, plays a vital role in maintaining a healthy gut. During sleep, the body undergoes essential repair and regeneration processes, including the restoration of the gut lining. Adequate sleep allows the gut microbiome to flourish and perform its vital functions. Disruptions in sleep patterns can lead to imbalances in the gut bacteria, potentially contributing to digestive issues.

Exercise and Gut Health

Physical activity is not only beneficial for our bodies but also for our gut. Exercise helps stimulate gut motility, promoting regular bowel movements. It can also reduce inflammation, which is often linked to gut disorders. Additionally, exercise can positively influence the composition of the gut microbiome, fostering a diverse and thriving ecosystem.

The Impact of Environmental Toxins

Our modern world is filled with an array of chemicals and pollutants that can negatively impact our health, including our gut. Pesticides, herbicides, and other environmental toxins can disrupt the delicate balance of the gut microbiome. Limiting exposure to these chemicals, when possible, and choosing organic foods can help protect gut health.

The Lesser Known Benefits of Grounding and Earthing

Grounding, or Earthing, involves connecting the body directly to the Earth's surface. This practice has gained attention for its potential health benefits, including improved sleep, reduced inflammation, and pain relief. While research is still emerging, some studies suggest that grounding may positively influence the gut microbiome by reducing oxidative stress.

The Lesser Known Role of Hydration in Gut Health

Hydration is often overlooked as a factor in gut health, but it plays a crucial role in maintaining optimal digestive function. Water helps to break down food, transport nutrients, and eliminate waste. Dehydration can lead to constipation and other digestive discomforts. Ensuring adequate hydration is essential for supporting a healthy gut.

Practical Exercise: Gut-Healing Smoothie

Ingredients:

- 1 cup spinach

- 1 banana

- 1/2 cup Greek yogurt

- 1/4 cup oats

- 1 tablespoon chia seeds

- 1/2 cup water

Instructions: Blend all ingredients until smooth. Enjoy daily: Incorporate this smoothie into your daily routine for a nutrient-rich and gut-friendly treat.

This smoothie is packed with fiber, probiotics, and antioxidants that can support gut health. The spinach provides essential nutrients, the banana adds sweetness, and the Greek yogurt offers protein and probiotics. The oats and chia seeds are excellent sources of fiber, which can help regulate digestion and promote a healthy gut microbiome.

Creating a Personalized Gut Health Plan

Embarking on a journey to optimize gut health and mental well-being is a deeply personal endeavor. There is no one-size-fits-all approach. Creating a personalized plan tailored to your unique needs and lifestyle is essential. Begin by assessing your current diet, exercise habits, stress levels, and sleep patterns. Identify areas for improvement and set realistic goals. Remember, small, consistent steps are often more effective than drastic changes.

Overcoming Challenges and Plateaus

The path to optimal gut health and mental well-being is rarely linear. You may encounter obstacles, setbacks, or plateaus along the way. It's important to view these challenges as opportunities for growth and learning. When faced with difficulties, reassess your plan, seek support, and stay patient. Remember, progress, not perfection, is the goal.

Tracking Your Progress: Tools and Techniques

Monitoring your progress is essential for staying motivated and making informed adjustments to your plan. There are various tools and techniques available to track your gut health and mental well-being. Food journals, mood trackers, and symptom diaries can provide valuable insights. Consider using wearable devices to monitor sleep patterns, heart rate variability, and other relevant metrics.

The Importance of Patience and Regularity

Transforming your gut health and mental well-being is a journey, not a sprint. Sustainable change takes time and consistency. Avoid quick fixes and fad diets.

Focus on building healthy habits that you can maintain in the long term. Celebrate small victories and be patient with yourself. Remember, progress, not perfection, is the ultimate goal.

The Lesser Known Role of Gut-Directed Therapies

In some cases, additional support may be necessary to address underlying gut imbalances. Gut-directed therapies, such as colonic hydrotherapy, probiotics, prebiotics, and fecal microbiota transplantation (FMT), have shown promise in treating certain gut disorders. However, these therapies should be considered under the guidance of a healthcare professional. It's essential to weigh the potential benefits and risks before proceeding.

Chapter 11: Nurturing Your Mind

Cognitive Health and Brain Function

The human brain is a marvel of complexity, a universe within itself. As we age, it's essential to nurture this intricate organ. Cognitive health, encompassing memory, attention, problem-solving, and learning, is the cornerstone of a fulfilling life. Engaging in mentally stimulating activities, such as puzzles, games, and learning new skills, can help preserve cognitive function and even enhance it.

Learning New Skills and Hobbies

The human mind is designed to learn and grow throughout life. Embracing new challenges and acquiring fresh skills not only keeps the mind sharp but also brings a sense of purpose and accomplishment. Whether it's learning a new language, taking up a musical instrument, or mastering a digital skill, the rewards are manifold. Engaging in stimulating activities can create new neural pathways, enhancing cognitive flexibility and resilience.

The Powers of Positive Thinking & Positive Transformation

Our thoughts are the architects of our reality. A positive mindset is not merely wishful thinking; it's a powerful tool for cultivating well-being. By focusing on the bright side and cultivating gratitude, we can reduce stress, boost our immune system, and improve our overall quality of life. Optimism is contagious, and it has the power to uplift not only ourselves but also those around us.

Whilst positive thinking is the beneficial practice of focusing on the bright side of life and maintaining an optimistic mindset, often involving the use of affirmations and a conscious effort to minimize negative thoughts, shifting your perspective to see opportunities rather than obstacles; Positive transformation, on the other hand, goes beyond mindset—it's more of a mindflow involving a holistic change in behavior, habits, and overall lifestyle.

While positive thinking can be a catalyst for positive transformation, the latter requires sustained action, self-discipline, and often, a deeper personal growth process that leads to tangible changes in one's life. Positive transformation is the result of applying positive thinking in a consistent and practical manner, leading to lasting improvements in various aspects of life.

Chapter 12: The Role of Community and Social Connection

Humans are inherently social creatures, and our connections with others are vital to our well-being. As we age, maintaining strong social connections becomes even more important. Social interaction provides emotional support, mental stimulation, and a sense of belonging. It can also help reduce feelings of loneliness and isolation, which can have a significant impact on our physical and mental health.

Building and maintaining strong relationships requires effort and intention. It involves active listening, empathy, and a willingness to be vulnerable. Cultivate meaningful connections with friends, family, and community members. Join clubs, groups, or organizations that align with your interests. Volunteering can be a rewarding way to meet new people and make a difference in your community.

Giving back to others can provide a sense of purpose and fulfillment. Volunteering your time and talents to a cause you care about can create a sense of belonging and connection. It can also boost your self-esteem and provide opportunities for personal growth.

Loneliness and isolation are common challenges among older adults. These feelings can have a detrimental impact on mental and physical health. To combat loneliness, reach out to others, join social activities, and explore new hobbies. Joining a senior center or community group can provide opportunities for social interaction and support.

The community plays a vital role in providing support and resources for older adults. Local organizations and government agencies often offer programs and services tailored to the needs of seniors. These may include transportation, meal delivery, social activities, and health care services. Connecting with community resources can help you access the support you need to age well.

By fostering strong social connections, engaging in volunteer work, and utilizing community resources, you can create a rich and fulfilling social life. These connections can provide emotional support, mental stimulation, and a sense of belonging, enhancing your overall well-being as you age.

Practical Exercise: Social Connection Inventory

- **Reflect on your social network**: Consider the quality and quantity of your relationships.

- **Identify areas for improvement:** Are there any social connections you'd like to strengthen or new ones you'd like to build?

- **Set goals**: Establish specific goals for enhancing your social connections, such as joining a club, volunteering, or reaching out to old friends.

- **Take action:** Start small and gradually increase your social activities. Attend events, join groups, or initiate conversations with new people.

- **Celebrate your progress:** Acknowledge your efforts and celebrate the positive changes in your social life.

This exercise can help you assess your current social connections and identify areas for improvement. By setting goals and taking action, you can create a more fulfilling and supportive social network. Remember, building strong relationships takes time and effort, but the rewards are immeasurable.

Building a Supportive Community

Surrounding yourself with a supportive community can significantly impact your journey to optimal health and mental well-being. Connect with like-minded individuals with similar goals. Sharing experiences, offering support, and learning from others can be invaluable. Online forums, support groups, and wellness communities can provide a sense of belonging and encouragement.

The Benefits of Social Connection

Humans are inherently social creatures, and our connections with others are vital to our mental and emotional health. Social interaction stimulates the brain, reduces loneliness, and provides a sense of belonging.

Sharing experiences, offering support, and receiving empathy from loved ones nourishes the soul. Building and maintaining strong social connections is essential for aging gracefully.

The Power of Positive Relationships

Strong social connections are essential for mental and physical health. Spending time with loved ones, friends, and community members can reduce stress, boost mood, and strengthen the immune system.

Practical Tip: Make time for social activities, such as joining clubs, volunteering, or simply spending time with friends and family.

Overcoming Loneliness and Isolation

Loneliness and isolation can have a negative impact on our well-being. To combat these feelings, it's important to reach out to others, join social groups, and engage in activities that bring joy.

Practical Tip: Consider volunteering, taking a class, or joining a book club to meet new people and connect with others who share your interests.

Embracing Solitude: The Benefits of Being Alone

While community and social connection are essential to well-being, there is also value in cultivating a healthy relationship with solitude. Spending time alone allows us to reconnect with ourselves, fostering resilience, creativity, and peace of mind. Embracing moments of solitude can deepen our understanding of who we are, clarify our thoughts, and give us the mental space needed to recharge.

The Benefits of Solitude

1. **Self-Reflection and Insight**: Time alone gives us the chance to reflect, process emotions, and gain insights into our experiences. This reflection promotes self-awareness, helping us understand our motivations, values, and goals.

2. **Increased Resilience and Independence:** By learning to find fulfillment in solitude, we strengthen our ability to face challenges on our own. This self-sufficiency fosters a sense of confidence, allowing us to navigate life's ups and downs with greater ease.

3. **Mental Clarity and Calm:** Solitude removes distractions, creating mental space to relax and quiet our thoughts. This time alone promotes clarity and calm, which can improve our mood and focus, making it easier to engage with others when we return to social settings.

Practical Exercises to Embrace Solitude

1. Mindful Breathing Practice

Set aside 5-10 minutes each day for quiet, mindful breathing. Sit in a comfortable spot, close your eyes, and focus on your breath. Notice each inhale and exhale, allowing your mind to settle. This brief practice calms the nervous system, helping you reconnect with yourself and find peace in solitude.

2. Going for Walks in Nature

Spend time alone in nature to experience the restorative effects of natural surroundings. As you walk, engage your senses fully: notice the colors, listen to the sounds around you, and feel the ground beneath your feet. Nature walks encourage relaxation and allow you to recharge while enhancing mindfulness and appreciation for the world around you.

3. Journaling for Reflection

Journaling is a powerful way to connect with your inner self. Spend a few minutes each day or week reflecting on your thoughts, emotions, and experiences. You could start with prompts like, "What am I grateful for today?" or "What brings me peace?" Over time, journaling helps you gain insight and provides a comforting routine for processing thoughts in solitude.

4. Practicing a "Digital Detox"

Take regular breaks from technology, even for an hour, to create uninterrupted time for yourself. During this time, focus on activities that don't involve screens, like reading, drawing, or simply sitting in silence. This practice encourages mental clarity and relaxation, helping you rediscover the benefits of slowing down and disconnecting.

Finding Balance Between Solitude and Social Connection

Solitude and connection are both vital aspects of a balanced life. By embracing moments of solitude, we build a solid foundation of self-awareness and resilience that enriches our relationships and helps us appreciate social interactions even more. When we learn to value both solitude and connection, we create a harmonious lifestyle that nurtures our mental and emotional well-being.

Chapter 13: Creating a Supportive Environment

Decluttering Your Physical and Mental Space

Our surroundings profoundly influence our well-being. A cluttered environment can mirror a cluttered mind, creating feelings of overwhelm and stress. Decluttering goes beyond mere aesthetics; it's a process of liberation. By letting go of physical possessions, we create space for new experiences and perspectives. This physical decluttering often mirrors an internal decluttering, allowing for mental clarity and focus.

The Importance of a Healthy Home Environment

Our homes are our sanctuaries, places of rest and rejuvenation. A healthy home environment is essential for supporting overall well-being. Good ventilation, adequate lighting, and proper temperature regulation contribute to physical comfort. Additionally, incorporating natural elements, such as plants or artwork inspired by nature, can create a soothing atmosphere. A home that nurtures the senses is a haven for the mind and body.

Building a Supportive Social Network

Humans are inherently social creatures, and our connections with others are vital to our happiness and longevity. Building and maintaining a strong social network provides emotional support, companionship, and a sense of belonging. Sharing experiences, offering help, and receiving support from others enriches our lives in countless ways. Investing time in relationships is an investment in our own well-being.

The Benefits of Nature Therapy

Spending time in nature has a profound impact on our mental and physical health. Forest bathing, gardening, and simply taking a walk in the park can reduce stress, improve mood, and boost creativity. Connecting with the natural world offers a sense of peace and perspective, allowing us to recharge and reconnect with ourselves.

The Lesser Known Role of Technology in Aging Well

Technology, often viewed as a disruptor, can also be a powerful tool for enhancing well-being in later life. From online communities and virtual connections to health monitoring devices and telemedicine, technology can bridge gaps, expand horizons, and improve quality of life. While it's essential to maintain a healthy balance, embracing technology can enrich the aging experience.

Practical Exercise: Digital Detox

1. **Choose a designated time**: Select a specific period, such as a weekend or a day off, for your digital detox.
2. **Disconnect from devices:** Turn off your phone, computer, and other electronic gadgets.
3. **Engage in offline activities:** Spend time in nature, read a book, practice a hobby, or connect with loved ones in person.
4. **Reflect on your experience:** After the digital detox, take some time to reflect on how you felt and what you learned.

A digital detox can help reduce stress, improve focus, and enhance your overall well-being. By disconnecting from technology, you can create space for mindfulness, relaxation, and meaningful connections.

Chapter 14: Financial Planning and Security

Budgeting and Saving Tips for Seniors

Effective financial planning is crucial for a secure retirement. Creating a budget, tracking expenses, and saving regularly can help you maintain financial stability.

Practical Tip: Consider using budgeting apps or spreadsheets to track your income and expenses.

Estate Planning and Inheritance

Estate planning is a crucial aspect of financial planning, especially for older adults. It involves creating a legal plan for the distribution of your assets after your death.

Key Considerations:

- **Will:** A legal document that outlines how your assets will be distributed.

- **Trust:** A legal arrangement that can be used to manage assets and minimize estate taxes.

- **Power of Attorney:** A legal document that authorizes someone to make decisions on your behalf.

Practical Tip: Consult with an estate planning attorney to create a personalized plan that meets your needs.

Long-Term Care Planning

As people age, the need for long-term care may arise. Long-term care insurance can help cover the costs of care, such as nursing home or home health aide services.

Practical Tip: Research long-term care insurance options and consider your specific needs and budget.

Medicare and Medicaid

Medicare and Medicaid are government programs that provide health insurance coverage to eligible individuals. Medicare is a federal program that provides health insurance for people aged 65 and older, as well as younger people with disabilities. Medicaid is a joint federal and state program that provides health coverage for low-income individuals and families.

Practical Tip: Consult with a healthcare professional or a Medicare advisor to understand your coverage options and maximize your benefits.

Chapter 15: Embracing Change and Adaptability

Change is an inevitable part of life, and it becomes even more pronounced as we age. Embracing change with resilience and adaptability is essential for navigating the challenges and opportunities that arise in later life.

Life transitions, such as retirement, health changes, or the loss of loved ones, can be significant sources of change. These transitions can bring both challenges and opportunities. By developing resilience and adaptability, we can navigate these changes with grace and find meaning and purpose in the process.

Resilience is the ability to bounce back from adversity and find strength in the face of challenges. It involves developing a positive mindset, cultivating emotional intelligence, and building strong social connections. By developing resilience, we can better cope with life's ups and downs and find meaning even in difficult times.

Adaptability is the capacity to adjust to new situations and circumstances. It involves being open to change, learning new skills, and embracing new experiences. By being adaptable, we can seize opportunities, overcome challenges, and continue to grow and evolve throughout our lives.

Letting go of the past can be challenging, but it is essential for embracing change and moving forward. Holding onto regrets or dwelling on the past can hinder our ability to live fully in the present. By letting go of the past, we can free ourselves from the burdens of the past and focus on creating a positive future.

Finding meaning and purpose in life transitions can be a powerful source of motivation and fulfillment. As we age, we may need to redefine our sense of purpose and find new ways to contribute to the world. Exploring new hobbies, volunteering, or pursuing personal goals can help us find meaning and purpose in our lives.

Practical Exercise: Reflection and Goal Setting

- **Reflect on your journey:** Take some time to reflect on the significant changes you've experienced in your life. Consider the challenges you've faced and the lessons you've learned.

- **Identify your values:** What is truly important to you? What brings you joy and fulfillment?

- **Set goals:** Based on your values, set goals for the future. These goals can be related to your health, relationships, career, or personal growth.

- **Create a vision:** Imagine your ideal future self. What does that person look like, feel like, and do?

- **Take action:** Start taking steps towards your goals, no matter how small. Celebrate your progress and stay focused on your vision.

By reflecting on your journey, identifying your values, and setting goals, you can create a sense of purpose and direction in your life. Embracing change and adaptability will empower you to navigate life's challenges with resilience, finding meaning and fulfillment in every stage of your journey.

Chapter 16: Spirituality and Meaning

Spirituality, often misunderstood as solely religious belief, is a broader concept that encompasses our connection to something greater than ourselves. It can provide a sense of meaning, purpose, and belonging, which are essential for aging well.

While spirituality can be expressed through religious practices, it doesn't have to be confined to a specific faith. Exploring different spiritual paths and beliefs can help you discover what resonates with you personally. Whether it's meditation, yoga, nature connection, or a formal religious practice, spirituality can offer a profound sense of peace and fulfillment.

Finding meaning and purpose in life is a fundamental human need. As we age, our sense of purpose may evolve, and it's essential to find new ways to contribute to the world and feel connected to something larger than ourselves. Volunteering, giving back to the community, and pursuing personal passions can all provide a sense of meaning and fulfillment.

Cultivating a sense of connection to something larger than oneself can offer solace, comfort, and a sense of belonging. This connection can be found through nature, community, spirituality, or a higher power. Whatever form it takes, this connection can provide a source of strength and resilience in the face of life's challenges.

Meditation, prayer, and mindfulness are powerful tools for cultivating spirituality and finding inner peace. These practices can help reduce stress, improve focus, and enhance our connection to ourselves and the world around us. By incorporating these practices into your daily life, you can deepen your sense of spirituality finding greater meaning and purpose.

Practical Exercise: Spiritual Reflection

1. **Find a quiet space:** Choose a place where you won't be disturbed.
2. **Reflect on your beliefs:** Consider your current beliefs about spirituality and meaning. Are there any changes you'd like to make?

3. **Explore different paths:** Research various spiritual practices and beliefs. Is there anything that resonates with you?
4. **Connect with others:** Share your spiritual journey with friends, family, or a spiritual community.
5. **Practice mindfulness:** Incorporate mindfulness meditation or other practices into your daily routine.

This exercise can help you explore your spirituality and find a path that resonates with you. Remember, spirituality is a personal journey, and there is no right or wrong way to practice it. The most important thing is to find what works for you and brings you a sense of peace and fulfillment.

Mindfulness Techniques for Stress Reduction

Mindfulness techniques can significantly reduce stress, improve focus, and enhance overall well-being. Beyond basic mindfulness meditation, there are several advanced practices to explore:

Body Scan Meditation: This technique involves systematically scanning your body, paying attention to each part and releasing any tension.

Loving-Kindness Meditation: This practice involves cultivating feelings of love, compassion, and kindness towards yourself and others.

Practical Tip: Designate a specific time each day for mindfulness practice, even if it's just for a few minutes.

The Power of Gratitude

Gratitude is a powerful tool for cultivating positive emotions and improving mental health. By focusing on the positive aspects of your life, you can increase your overall happiness and well-being.

Practical Tip: Keep a gratitude journal and write down three things you're grateful for each day.

Finding Meaning and Purpose in Later Life

Finding meaning and purpose in life can enhance your overall well-being and longevity. Here are some strategies to help you discover your purpose:

- **Volunteer:** Give back to your community and help others.

- **Learn a new skill:** Take up a new hobby or learn a new language.

- **Connect with nature:** Spend time outdoors and appreciate the beauty of the natural world.

- **Practice mindfulness:** Cultivate a sense of peace and presence in your daily life.

- **Build strong relationships:** Nurture your relationships with loved ones and friends.

By incorporating these practices into your daily life, you can enhance your overall well-being and live a more fulfilling life.

Epilogue

Aging is not a destination but a journey. It is a chapter filled with unique challenges and extraordinary opportunities. This book has highlighted key principles for navigating this journey with grace, resilience, and vitality.

Throughout these pages, we have delved into the intricate relationship between mind and body, understanding how our thoughts, emotions, and behaviors can profoundly influence our physical health. We have explored the importance of nourishing our bodies, expanding our minds, cultivating a supportive environment, finding meaning, purpose in life, and more.

Plus, this book is more than just information. It is a practical guide, filled with actionable advice and exercises to help you implement these principles in your daily life. By incorporating biohacking, mindful breathing, mindful eating, chair yoga, gut-healing smoothies, gratitude journaling, digital detoxes, social connection exercises, reflection, goal setting, and spiritual practices into your routine, you can take tangible steps towards improving your well-being.

Remember, there is no one-size-fits-all approach to aging well. Each individual's journey is unique. The key is to create a personalized mind-body plan that resonates with your passions, values, and lifestyle. Experiment with different practices, listen to your body, and celebrate your progress. It's about embracing the process, celebrating your accomplishments, and learning from your challenges. By understanding the mind-body connection and taking proactive steps to nurture both, you can unlock the full potential of your later years.

Aging is not about clinging to the past but embracing the present and envisioning a vibrant future. It is a time for reflection, growth, and giving back. Let us redefine aging as a period of wisdom, creativity, and purpose. By embracing the aging process as a natural and beautiful part of life, we unlock the potential for a truly extraordinary journey.

Let's embark on this journey together. Age well, live fully, and embrace the beauty of the aging process.

Your adventure resumes.

I hope you found this book beneficial and will put the information to good use. Remember, the journey to aging well is a personal one. Take the time to reflect on your own experiences and tailor the guidance in this book to your specific needs and goals.

* * *

Thank you so much for making it all the way!

I greatly value the time you shared with my book. As a small Indie publisher it means a lot, and I hope I'm making a difference in your Aging Well Journey.

If you have 60 seconds, reading your honest feedback on the site you got it from, would mean the world to me! It does wonders for the book, and I love learning about your experience with it.

So if you've had a positive experience with *Age Well, Live Fully: Your Mind-Body Prescription*, please take a moment to leave a review. Your feedback helps me to improve, and serve more patrons like you.

Chris

***

Most Frequently Asked Questions

Q: How can I stay motivated to maintain a healthy lifestyle as I age?

A: Maintaining motivation can be challenging, but it's essential for aging well. Here are a few tips:

- **Set realistic goals:** Break down larger goals into smaller, achievable steps.
- **Find a workout buddy:** Having a workout partner can help you stay accountable.
- **Mix up your routine:** Try different activities to keep things interesting.
- **Reward yourself:** Celebrate your accomplishments, no matter how small.
- **Focus on the positive:** Remind yourself of the benefits of a healthy lifestyle.

Q: What can I do to improve my mental health as I age?

A: Prioritizing mental health is crucial at any age. Here are some tips:

- **Practice mindfulness:** Engage in activities like meditation or yoga to reduce stress and improve focus.
- **Connect with others:** Maintain strong social relationships to combat loneliness and isolation.
- **Challenge your mind:** Learn new skills, read books, or play games to keep your mind sharp.
- **Seek professional help if needed:** Don't hesitate to talk to a therapist or counselor.

Q: How can I adapt to changes in my body as I age?

A: As we age, our bodies undergo natural changes. Here are some tips for adapting to these changes:

- **Listen to your body:** Pay attention to your body's signals and adjust your activities accordingly.
- **Stay active:** Regular exercise can help maintain strength, flexibility, and balance.
- **Eat a healthy diet:** A balanced diet can help you maintain a healthy weight and support your overall health.
- **Get enough sleep:** Aim for 7-9 hours of quality sleep each night.

Q: How can I maintain a positive outlook on aging?

A: A positive outlook on aging can significantly impact your overall well-being. Here are some tips for staying positive:

- **Focus on the present moment:** Don't dwell on the past or worry about the future.
- **Practice gratitude:** Take time to appreciate the good things in your life.
- **Surround yourself with positive people:** Spend time with people who uplift and inspire you.
- **Cultivate a sense of humor:** Laughter can help reduce stress and improve your mood.

By incorporating these tips into your daily routine, you can age gracefully and live a fulfilling life.

Don't miss out!

Visit the website below and you can sign up to receive emails whenever Chris Josinlah publishes a new book. There's no charge and no obligation.

https://books2read.com/r/B-A-KJIQC-QWWGF

BOOKS 2 READ

Connecting independent readers to independent writers.

Did you love *Age Well, Live Fully: Your Mind-Body Prescription*? Then you should read *The Minimalist Monk's Guide to a Clutter-Free Life: Zen Approach to a Tidy Home & Mind*[1] by Chris Josinlah!

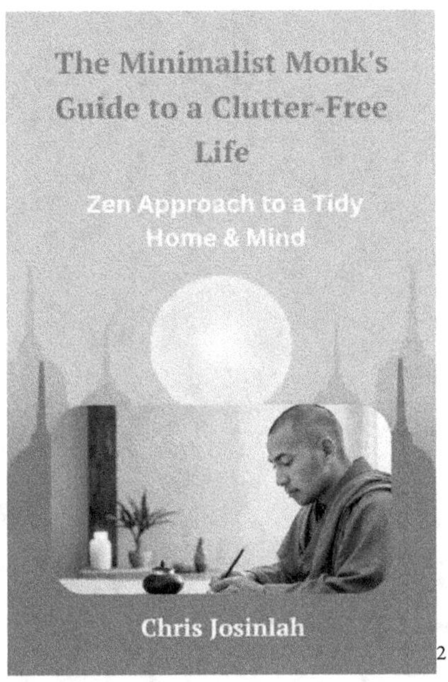

[2]

Tired of feeling overwhelmed by clutter? Ready to simplify your life and find inner peace?

The Minimalist Monk's Guide to a Clutter-Free Life is your ultimate guide to a serene and organized home. Inspired by ancient wisdom, this book combines practical decluttering techniques with mindfulness practices to help you:

Declutter Your Space: Organize your home, office, and digital life.**Declutter Your Mind:** Reduce stress and anxiety through mindfulness.**Simplify Your Life:** Adopt a minimalist lifestyle and focus on what truly matters.

Imagine the freedom and clarity that comes with a clutter-free environment. This book will help you:

Increase Productivity: A clutter-free space leads to a clear mind.**Improve Your Mental Health:** Reduce stress and anxiety.**Enhance Your Creativity:** A serene

---

1. https://books2read.com/u/4NqLOz

2. https://books2read.com/u/4NqLOz

environment sparks inspiration.

Take the first step towards a more peaceful and organized life. Order your copy of *The Minimalist Monk's Guide to a Clutter-Free Life* today!

Also by Chris Josinlah

The Minimalist Monk's Guide to a Clutter-Free Life: Zen Approach to a Tidy
Home & Mind
Age Well, Live Fully: Your Mind-Body Prescription